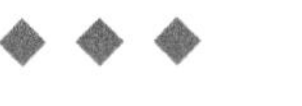 

Copyright ©2020 LISA H. GREGORY PH.D

CONTENTS

INTRODUCTION

Protein is an important nutrient for weight loss. Getting enough can boost your metabolism, reduce your appetite and help you lose body fat without losing muscle.

Protein shakes are an easy way to add more protein to your diet, and have been shown to help with weight loss.

This book explains everything you need to know about protein shakes and how they affect your weight.

WHAT ARE PROTEIN SHAKES?

Protein shakes are drinks made by mixing protein powder with water, although other ingredients are often added as well.

They can be a convenient addition to the diet, especially when access to quality high-protein foods is limited.

Although most people don't need them to meet daily protein requirements, they can also be useful if you need to increase your intake for some reason.

You can buy protein powder and mix it yourself, but you can also get many different brands of pre-made liquid shakes.

Some of the most popular types of protein powder on the market are:

• Whey protein: Quickly absorbed, dairy-based. Contains all the essential amino acids.

• Casein protein: Slowly absorbed, dairy-based. Contains all essential amino acids

• Soy protein: Plant-based and contains all essential amino acids. Also contains soy isoflavones, which may provide some health benefits.

• Hemp protein: Plant-based and high in omega-3 and

omega-6 fats, but low in the essential amino acid lysine.

• Rice protein: Plant-based and low in the essential amino acid lysine.

• Pea protein: Plant-based and low in the non-essential amino acids cystine and methionine.

Some brands contain a mix of different types of protein powder. For example, many plant-based brands combine types to complement each other's amino acid profile.

Bottom line:
Protein shakes can contain different types of protein, each with its own characteristics.

Want some protein shakes you'll actually ENJOY drinking? I've made a list of all the Best Low Carb Protein Shakes just for you. These are all perfect for Keto and low-carb diets and are SO good!

BEST LOW CARB PROTEIN SHAKES

Why do I call these the Best Low carb Protein Shakes? Well, not only are they yummy, but I show you to how to make low carb or keto protein shakes that you can customize by doing a mix and match with some basic ingredients. So don't just follow a recipe, learn how to make your own low carb protein shakes.

Don't limit these to just breakfast time. I often have one of these for a meal. Just watch the carb counts by entering in a recipe into your tracker BEFORE you make it! Otherwise, you may be in for an unpleasant surprise.

BEST SMOOTHIE RECIPES

Eating low-carb can be frustrating. If you're new to eating Keto or low carb, you can struggle with all the foods you're "missing out" on and feel deprived. Feeling deprived can lead to cravings and cheating and you don't want to go down that road. The way you can avoid all those things is by being prepared and having a plan.

One big way I shake off cravings and a sweet tooth is by utilizing this list of the Best Low Carb Smoothie recipes. They're filling, high in protein and perfect if you're on a full liquid diet. They will satisfy that sweet tooth in a healthy way. Outside of that, they're so easy to just throw in the blender and make!

HOW TO MAKE THE BEST LOW CARB PROTEIN SHAKES FOR YOU

Making low carb protein shakes is a lot easier than you think. You start by selecting a liquid, a source of protein, a source of fat, and some flavorings. So let's talk about each of these, and what choices you have available to you.

You may want to play around with these meal replacement shakes to suit your taste buds. But as a starting point:

Proportions for These Protein Shakes

1. Add Protein

1/4 cup protein such as cottage cheese, yogurt, etc.

2. Pour In Liquid

1 cup liquid such as hemp milk, almond milk, etc.

3. Add Fat

1 tablespoon fat such as peanut butter, coconut oil, etc.

4. Season Well

1/2 teaspoons of seasonings such as cinnamon, nutmeg, etc.

5. Add Ice To Your Liking

1 cup ice.

6. Mix In A High Powered Blender

Put all this into a high power blender (I use this one) and whirl away!

LIQUIDS FOR MAKING THE BEST LOW CARB PROTEIN SHAKE RECIPES FOR YOU

There is no reason at all why you should not use plain water. If you have enough flavors in the rest of your ingredients, then water may be your best option. If you'd rather use something else, here are a few things to consider:

• Almond milk, hemp milk, or coconut milk in cartons (low carb, unsweetened, good taste). Do not use rice milk as it tends to be high in carbs.

• Heavy Whipping cream (lots of calories so use sparingly)

• Half and half (little heavier on carbs)

• High protein lactose-free milk like Fairlife (higher carbs so monitor carefully)

• Canned coconut milk (lots of calories so use sparingly)

SOURCES OF PROTEIN FOR THE BEST LOW CARB PROTEIN SHAKES

I've used protein powders for 5 years now and love Syntrax protein. But there are some other sources for protein that you should also consider in your low carb protein shake recipes.

• Greek yogurt (watch the carb count)

• Tofu (no you won't be able to taste tofu in there)

• Cottage cheese

• Variety of protein powders that you like. This is the best way to add a lot of flavor. Take for example banana protein powder. Bananas are not low carb. But if you really want a banana strawberry smoothie, you can have one--as long as you use banana protein powder.

SOURCES OF FAT FOR THE BEST LOW CARB PROTEIN SHAKES

The easiest ones here for me are various nut butters. Not only do they make the protein drinks thicker and tastier, but they're an easy way to add some fat to your diet. Here are a few options to consider.

• All types of nut butters such as almond butter, peanut butter (no sugar added, watch the carbs)

• Avocado. This is actually a very creamy addition to your shake. I know we think of Avocado as savory in the United States, but I've had some amazing sweet avocado shakes in Vietnam, and I highly recommend this.

• Straight up butter, MCT oil, or coconut oil. I've not had the best luck with butter and coconut oil as they tend to clump in a cold shake, but MCT oil in small quantities works well for me.

• Whole nuts. If you don't want to worry about the added sugar and salt in store-bought nut butters, just had nuts directly into your healthy smoothie recipe or protein shake and let the blender do the job for you.

SOURCES OF FLAVORINGS FOR THE BEST PROTEIN SHAKES

• Spices. My favorite way to add flavor to shakes and to make the same combination of ingredients taste different from day to day. I often use cardamom, cinnamon, nutmeg, small amounts of cloves, or ready mixes like pumpkin pie spice or apple pie spice to add sweetness to my low carb protein shakes. These are the easiest since you're adding no carbs, protein, fat, etc., just yummy flavor. You will soon learn what types of spiced low carb protein shakes you like best.

• Fruits. Here's an area you really need to be careful. While fruit has its place in a low carb protein shake, only certain types of fruits will work, and even then, only in small quantities. You can use all types of berries, but I would urge you to never use more than 1/3 of a cup of berries at most. I often use frozen berries as they not only cool the drink immediately, but they're also easier to store. If you're only going to be using a few berries here and there, it's hard to do this with fresh berries.

• Sugar-free Flavored Syrups. A quick search for sugar-free flavored syrups will show you the various options at your disposal including chocolate syrup, peppermint, hazelnut, caramel etc. I haven't included these in the shakes above because I prefer to get flavor from real food, but these sugar-free syrups are a very popular option for flavoring low carb protein shakes.

Just remember, the Best Low Carb Protein Shake is one that YOU like. So start with these protein shake recipes and play around until you get what you have your own best low carb protein shake. Also, don't limit these to just breakfast time. I often have one of these for a meal replacement. Just watch the carb counts by entering in a recipe into your tracker BEFORE you make it! Otherwise, you may be in for an unpleasant surprise.

BEST LOW-CARB, KETO-FRIENDLY PROTEIN POWDERS

From weight loss to better blood sugar control to healthy aging, the benefits of protein are well established.

While you can likely meet your protein needs through your diet, protein powders offer a convenient and easy way to increase your intake.

Many people following low-carb or ketogenic diets turn to protein powders to supplement their diet.

However, choosing the right one to fit your low-carb or keto lifestyle can be challenging due to the countless forms and sources of protein powder.

That said, several types are particularly low in carbs and make superb choices for anyone monitoring their carb intake.

7 BEST LOW-CARB, KETO-FRIENDLY PROTEIN POWDERS.

1. Whey Protein Isolate

Whey protein is one of two proteins derived from dairy.

Owing to its amino acid profile, whey protein is a high-quality source of protein that your body can digest and absorb quickly.

The two main types of whey protein are concentrate and isolate.

During the manufacturing process of whey protein powder, much of the lactose — or milk sugar — is filtered out, leaving a condensed product called whey protein concentrate.

Whey protein concentrate contains 35–80% protein by weight. For instance, a typical scoop of 80% whey protein by weight will contain about 25 grams of protein and 3–4 grams of carbs — and, if flavoring is added, possibly more

Whey protein concentrate is then further processed and filtered to make an even more concentrated product called whey protein isolate, which boasts 90–95% protein by weight.

Whey protein isolates have the highest percentage of pure protein and the lowest number of carbs per serving of any whey protein.

Summary
Whey protein isolate is the purest form of whey protein you can buy. It contains few — or even zero — carbohydrates per scoop.

2. Casein Protein
Casein, the other milk protein, is also high in quality but digested and absorbed much more slowly by your body than whey.

This makes casein protein ideal for periods of fasting, such as before bed or between meals.

Like its whey counterpart, casein powder undergoes processing that extracts carbs and fat, leaving a concentrated source of protein

Both Dymatize and NutraBio make a casein protein powder that provides only 2 grams of carbs and 25 grams of protein per 36-gram and 34-gram scoop, respectively.

Casein powders not only offer few carbs and generous amounts of protein but are a good source of calcium, an important mineral your body needs for bone health, muscle contractions and blood clotting.

For instance, the products from Dymatize and NutraBio boast 70% of the Daily Value (DV) for calcium per scoop.

Use more water to mix casein powder than you would with whey, as casein tends to thicken when stirred.

Summary

Casein is a milk protein that your body digests slowly. Protein powder made from casein provides few carbs and a good amount of calcium.

3. Egg Protein

Eggs are one of the most nutritious foods you can eat.

They're packed with protein, essential vitamins and minerals and other important nutrients like choline, which is important for proper brain and nervous system functioning.

Egg-white protein powders are manufactured by removing the yolks and dehydrating the remaining egg whites, turning them into powder.

The egg whites are also pasteurized to deactivate avidin, a protein that inhibits the absorption of biotin, a crucial B vitamin.

Since egg whites naturally hold trivial amounts of carbs and fat, egg-white protein powders are a good option if you're following a low-carb diet.

MRM makes a quality egg-white protein powder that provides 2 grams of carbs and 23 grams of protein or the equivalent of six egg whites per scoop (33 grams).

Some egg protein powders include both the white and yolk — which contains most of the important nutrients in eggs.

This egg-yolk protein powder from KetoThin boasts a good amount of fat — 15 grams — and a moderate amount of protein — 12 grams — with just 1 gram of carbs per scoop (30 grams), making it a perfect keto protein powder.

Egg-yolk protein powders do contain a relatively high amount of cholesterol, which was long thought to raise cholesterol levels in your body and contribute to heart disease.

However, research suggests that dietary cholesterol has little to no effect on blood cholesterol levels in most people. Thus, there is no significant link between the cholesterol you eat and your risk of heart disease.

Summary
Egg protein powder is an excellent choice if you follow a low-carb or keto diet. Egg-white protein powder contains only the protein from the white, whereas whole-egg protein powder includes the white alongside the yolk.

4. Collagen Protein
Collagen is the most common structural protein in your body. It's primarily found in your hair, skin, nails, bones, ligaments and tendons.

Collagen's unique composition of amino acids gives it many purported health benefits, such as promoting body composition in older adults, as well as healthy skin and joints.

However, collagen lacks one of the essential amino acids that your body needs for good health. Because your body can't make essential amino acids, it must get them from your diet.

Collagen protein powder, also called collagen peptides, is made from animal byproducts — usually cowhide, cow bones, chicken bones, eggshell membranes and fish scales.

Most available collagen protein powders are tasteless and

unflavored, making them great to stir into soups or drinks like coffee.

What's more, they're naturally carb-free.

Vital Proteins makes a beef collagen product that contains 0 carbs and 17 grams of protein for every two scoops (20 grams), while Sports Research offers a similar product with 0 carbs and 10 grams of protein per scoop (11 grams).

Many flavored collagen protein powders are fortified with medium-chain triglycerides (MCTs), which are fats found in foods like coconut oil.

MCTs are easily digested and absorbed, providing your body with an alternative source of fuel particularly when you severely restrict carbs, as with the keto diet.

For instance, one scoop (17 grams) of this product by Perfect Keto offers 1 gram of carbs, 10 grams of protein and 4 grams of fat from MCTs.

Summary
Collagen protein powders, which are derived from the connective tissues of animals and fish, may offer unique health benefits. Some are fortified with MCTs, which benefit those following a keto diet.

5. Soy Protein Isolate
Soybeans are a type of legume that's naturally high in protein.

Soy protein powder is created by grinding soybeans into a meal and then into soy protein isolate, which consists of 90–95% protein by weight and is practically free of carbs.

Keep in mind that manufacturers sometimes add sugar and flavorings that can contribute unwanted carbs.

For example, this vanilla-flavored soy protein isolate product by NOW Sports holds 13 grams of carbs and 25 grams of protein per scoop (45 grams).

A better option is this unflavored product by the same company, which has 0 carbs and 20 grams of protein per scoop (24 grams).

Summary

Because it's naturally high in protein, soy makes for a great protein powder. Unflavored powders have almost no carbs and are packed with protein, though flavored varieties may be higher in carbs due to added sugars and flavorings.

6. Pea Protein Isolate

Peas are another type of legume that naturally contains a sizable amount of protein (29 Trusted Source).

Similar to soy protein isolate, pea protein powder is made by grinding dried peas into a powder and extracting the carbs, leaving an isolated powder.

Manufacturers frequently add sugar — and therefore carbs — to increase palatability.

For example, this flavored pea protein isolate from NOW Sports packs 9 grams of carbs with 24 grams of protein per scoop (44 grams).

On the other hand, one scoop (33 grams) of the unflavored version contains just 1 gram of carbs alongside 24 grams of protein.

Summary

Pea protein powder, which is very low in carbs, offers you a great protein boost — but watch out for flavored varieties, as these often harbor more carbs.

7. Rice Protein Isolate

Rice protein is a popular plant-based protein, particularly because it's hypoallergenic — meaning it's unlikely to cause allergic reactions.

Most rice protein powders contain 80% of protein by weight, less than that of soy or pea protein.

While rice is particularly rich in carbs, rice protein powder is typically made by treating brown rice with enzymes that cause the carbs to separate from the proteins.

For instance, this chocolate-flavored rice protein powder product from NutriBiotic contains just 2 grams of carbs but 11 grams of protein per heaping tablespoon (16 grams).

The same company also offers a plain rice protein powder with 2 grams of carbs and 12 grams of protein per heaping tablespoon (15 grams).

Summary
Rice protein powder is surprisingly low-carb because the carbs in this common grain are extracted from the proteins.

HOW TO ADD FLAVOR TO UNFLAVORED PRODUCTS

If you spring for an unflavored animal- or plant-based protein powder, there are several ways to make them tastier.

These include:

• Add small amounts of cocoa powder.

• Stir the powder into low-calorie beverages like almond milk or powdered drink mixes.

• Drizzle in sugar-free syrups.

• Spoon in artificial sweeteners like Splenda or natural sweeteners, including stevia or monk fruit extract.

• Mix small amounts of unflavored protein powder with soups, stews or oatmeal.

• Stir in sugar-free, flavored pudding mixes.

• Add natural flavor extracts or spices, such as cinnamon.

Summary

Zing up your unflavored protein powders with sweeteners and spices, or try adding them to various dishes.

The Bottom Line

Protein powders are an easy and versatile way to supplement your diet.

Many are inherently low in carbs since they're extracted during the manufacturing process.

The milk proteins — whey and casein — and egg proteins are some of the best low-carb and keto-friendly protein powders, while collagen proteins typically contain no carbs but have less protein than whey or egg varieties.

Plant-based protein powders made from soy, peas or rice also make an excellent fit for a low-carb lifestyle.

While flavored versions of these powders often harbor more carbs, unflavored versions contain almost none.

All in all, it's easy to select from several protein powders to optimize your low-carb or keto diet based on your preferences and goals.

HOW PROTEIN SHAKES HELP YOU LOSE WEIGHT AND BELLY FAT

Protein Shakes Decrease Hunger and Appetite

Protein can decrease hunger and appetite in two main ways.

• First, it increases levels of appetite-reducing hormones like GLP-1, PYY and CCK, while reducing levels of the hunger hormone ghrelin.

• Second, protein helps you feel full for longer.

In one study, a high-protein breakfast helped participants consume up to 135 fewer calories later in the day.

In another, overweight men who had been on a weight loss diet increased their protein intake to 25% of total calories. This increase cut cravings by 60% and late-night snacking by half.

Increasing protein intake from 15% to 30% of total calories helped participants in another study consume 441 fewer calories per day without actively trying to limit their portions.

What's more, by the end of the 12-week study period, they had lost an average of 11 lbs (5 kg).

These shakes can be a convenient way to add extra protein to your diet. However, keep in mind that too much can still lead to excess calories.

Another study found that shakes containing 20-80 grams of protein all decreased hunger by 50-65%, regardless of the amount of protein in their shakes.

So if you're trying to lose weight, 20 grams per shake seems sufficient to reduce hunger.

Bottom line:
Protein can decrease your appetite by affecting your hunger hormones. It can also help you feel full for longer, which can help you eat less and lose body fat.

PROTEIN SHAKES MAY INCREASE METABOLISM

High protein intake can boost your metabolism, helping you burn slightly more calories each day.

That's in part because a high-protein diet — especially when combined with strength training — may help you build muscle.

This can speed up your metabolism because muscle burns more calories than fat.

One study gave obese participants shakes with either 200 or 0 grams of extra protein per week.

Those given the protein gained 2.8 lbs (1.3 kg) more mass following a 13-week training program.

In another study, researchers gave participants a combination of foods and shakes providing either 0.5 g/lbs or 1.1 g/lbs (1.2 g/kg or 2.4 g/kg) of protein per day.

After 6 weeks, those on the higher-protein diet gained 2.4 lbs (1.1 kg) more muscle and lost 2.9 lbs (1.3 kg) more fat.

It should be noted, however, that your ability to gain muscle during a weight loss diet may depend on the amount of muscle you already have.

Protein can also increase metabolism because of the amount of calories needed to digest and metabolize it. This is known as the thermic effect of food (TEF).

For instance, 15-30% of protein calories are burned during digestion, while only 5-10% of carb calories and 0-3% of fat calories are burned during digestion.

Bottom line:
Protein helps boost metabolism because a lot of energy is spent digesting and metabolizing it. It also helps you build muscle, which burns more calories than fat.

PROTEIN SHAKES MAY HELP YOU LOSE WEIGHT AND BELLY FAT

Researchers generally agree that high-protein diets can help you lose more fat, especially fat from the belly area.

In one study, participants on a diet providing 25% of calories as protein lost 10% more belly fat after 12 months than those eating half that amount.

In another, participants given an extra 56 grams of whey protein per day had lost 5 lbs (2.3 kg) more at the end of a 23-week study period, despite not consciously changing anything else in their diet.

A separate study compared the effect of various weight loss diets. The participants consuming more protein lost 31 lbs (14.1 kg) in 3 months — 23% more than those consuming less.

In one final study, participants on diets providing 30% of calories from protein lost 8.1 lbs (3.7 kg) more than those on diets providing 15% of calories from protein.

Bottom line:

Protein shakes are a convenient way to increase your daily protein intake. This can help boost fat loss, especially from around your mid-section.

PROTEIN SHAKES MAY ALSO PREVENT MUSCLE LOSS AND METABOLIC SLOWDOWN

Weight loss diets often cause you to lose muscle, which can slow down your metabolism. This makes it easier to gain all the weight back (and more) once you go off the diet.

A high protein intake combined with strength training can help prevent part of this muscle loss and metabolic slowdown.

In fact, researchers reported that participants' metabolism decreased less on a weight loss diet providing 36% of calories as protein than on a diet providing about half that amount (30Trusted Source).

Evidence shows that consuming a daily protein shake as part of a weight loss diet may make muscle maintenance up to three and a half times more efficient.

A study of athletes compared weight loss diets providing

either 35% or 15% of calories from protein. Both diets helped participants lose about the same amount of fat, but those consuming more protein lost 38% less muscle mass.

A recent review further notes that weight loss diets that exceed 0.5 g/lbs (1.0 g/kg) of protein per day can help older adults retain more muscle and lose more fat.

Bottom line:
Protein shakes consumed during a weight loss diet can help prevent muscle loss and metabolic slowdown. This is particularly effective in combination with strength training.

PROTEIN SHAKES MAY HELP PREVENT WEIGHT RE-GAIN AFTER WEIGHT LOSS

Protein's effect on metabolism, appetite and muscle mass may also keep you from regaining the fat you worked so hard to lose.

One study reports that participants given more protein lost more weight and maintained their results better than those given less.

In fact, the high-protein group regained only 9% of the lost weight, whereas the low-protein group regained 23%.

Another study gave participants who just completed a weight loss intervention a supplement that provided 48.2 grams of protein per day.

Participants who took the supplement felt fuller after meals and had regained 50% less weight 6 months later, compared to those given no supplement.

A separate study noted similar effects with a supplement that provided only 30 grams of protein per day, once again showing that more is not necessarily better.

Bottom line:
Additional protein, whether from shakes or whole foods, can help minimize the amount of weight you regain after weight loss.

WHICH TYPE OF PROTEIN IS BEST?

Different types of protein have different effects on the body.

For instance, whey is more quickly absorbed than casein, helping you feel less hungry in the short-term.

One study reports that 56 grams of whey protein per day helped overweight and obese participants lose 5 lbs (2.3 kg) more fat than the same amount of soy protein.

Another describes whey as 3 times more effective at maintaining muscle-building ability during a weight loss diet than soy protein.

That being said, not all studies agree that whey is superior. For example, one report notes that the faster hunger-reducing effect results in no differences in the amount of calories consumed at meals.

Furthermore, several reviews report equal amounts of fat loss with use of whey, soy, rice or egg-protein supplements.

One final factor to consider is the protein's quality.

Whey, casein and soy contain all the essential amino acids your body needs.

On the other hand, rice and hemp protein are low in the essential amino acid lysine, and pea protein is also low in the non-essential amino acids cystine and methionine.

That being said, these deficiencies likely don't cause a problem unless if shakes are the only source of protein in your diet.

Also, many plant-based protein powders mix different sources so that the mixture contains all the essential amino acids.

Bottom line:
The exact type of protein powder you have in your shakes should not make a major difference for fat loss. Some studies show an advantage for whey, but the evidence is mixed.

DOSAGE AND SIDE EFFECTS

Taking 1 shake per day should be a good way to start.

It is best to take it either before or instead of a meal, with 1 or 2 scoops of protein powder in the shake.

Mixing it with water, ice and perhaps a piece of fruit in a blender is a simple way to create a delicious and satisfying shake.

Side effects such as bloating, cramps, gas and diarrhea may occur if you're lactose intolerant and drinking shakes made with whey or casein.

These symptoms can be simply avoided by switching to protein powders not derived from dairy, such as egg, pea, soy, hemp or rice protein powders.

Of note, high-protein diets were once thought to have negative impacts on kidney and bone health, but newer research shows this is not true.

In fact, high protein intakes were never shown to cause any kidney damage in healthy people. However, lower-protein diets may be beneficial for those with existing kidney issues.

Protein is also an essential nutrient for bone formation and maintenance, and reviews show that there is no reason to restrict your intake to improve bone health.

Most studies report that total protein intakes of between 0.5-1.0 g/lbs (1.2-2.2 g/kg) per day provide most beneficial effects for weight loss.

This amount of protein normally represents around 25-35% of the calories you consume in one day and is generally considered safe.

Bottom line:
Taking one shake per day is a good way to start, with 1 or 2 scoops of protein. Some people may experience digestive side effects.

22 BEST PROTEIN SHAKE RECIPES FOR WEIGHT LOSS

Boost calorie burn and satiety while preserving lean muscle mass with these high protein shakes ready at the push of a button.

Packed with essential nutrients that keep your skin, hair, bones, muscles healthy, there's virtually no prep work or cleanup with protein shakes. But not just any drink will do. Protein sips from local gyms and juice shops often carry more added sugar than a dozen donuts and the same holds true for some recipes you'll find on the web. Sorry to say, slugging those back every day won't get you any closer to your body goals. That is, of course, unless you choose from our round-up of the healthiest protein shake recipes.

To help you stay on track, we searched the web for the most mouth-watering protein shake recipes for weight loss out there. Below, you'll find something to satisfy every craving from refreshingly fruity to a milkshake-inspired dessert. Since we've taken care of finding the nutritional winners, all you have to do is pick a recipe, start up the blender and enjoy.

To build muscle, lose weight, or just feel fuller, enjoy these

22 best protein shake recipes.

1. Fresh Blueberry Smoothie (28 g protein)
Blueberry banana protein shake recipe

Nutrition: 232 calories, 6 g fat, 16 g carbs, 3 g fiber, 28 g protein

½ cup unsweetened almond milk

1 scoop vanilla plant-based protein powder

½ cup frozen blueberries

½ tbsp natural unsalted almond butter

Water to blend (optional)

2. Peanut Butter Cup Shake (30 g protein)
Peanut butter banana smoothie

Nutrition: 258 calories, 6 g fat, 21 g carbs, 5 g fiber, 30 g protein

Protein Source: protein powder

½ cup unsweetened almond milk

1 scoop vanilla or chocolate plant-based protein powder

1 tbsp. unsweetened cocoa powder

½ frozen banana

½ tbsp. natural unsalted peanut butter

Water to blend (optional)

3. Vanilla Chai Shake (19 g protein)

Banana almond butter smoothie

Nutrition: 219 calorie, 9 g fat, 20 g carbs, 4 g fiber, 17 g protein

Protein Source: protein powder

¼ cup unsweetened almond milk

¼ cup chai tea (brewed from a teabag and chilled)

1 scoop plant-based vanilla protein powder

½ frozen banana

¼ tsp. ground cinnamon

½ tbsp. unsalted natural almond butter

Water to blend (optional)

4. Green Monster (15 g protein)
Nutrition: 271 calories, 6 g fat, 40 g carbs, 8 g fiber, 15 g protein

Protein Source: protein powder

¼ cup no-sugar-added apple juice

¼ cup water

1 scoop plant-based vanilla protein powder

½ Bosc pear, chopped

½ cup baby spinach, loosely packed

¼ ripe avocado

½ frozen banana

5. Peanut Butter and Jelly Protein Smoothie (16 g protein)

Nutrition: 228 calories, 7.5 g fat, 1.3 g saturated fat, 23 g carbs, 5 g fiber, 11 g sugar, 16 g protein

Protein Source: Soy milk, peanut butter, and protein powder

If you're a big fan of the classic childhood sandwich, you've got to give this recipe a try it's like sipping a little bit of salty-sweet heaven through a straw. Blending frozen berries with all-natural peanut butter, vanilla protein, rolled oats, and soy milk helps create the protein-packed delicious taste without tons of excess calories. If you're not a fan of soy milk, feel free to sub in any type of unsweetened milk you prefer. It won't alter the taste or nutrition profile much.

6. Spinach Flax Protein Smoothie (19 g protein)

Nutrition: 231 calories, 8 g fat, 0 g saturated fat, 23 g carbs, 9 g fiber, 11 g sugar, 19 g protein

Protein Source: Optional protein powder, flax meal, chia seeds

This is the spinach smoothie for people who don't like spinach but want to. Thanks to the addition of mango, pineapple, and banana, you won't even taste the leafy green but you'll still reap all of its health benefits. In fact, this drink serves up 33 percent of the day's vitamin A most of which comes from the leaves. The addition of chia seeds and flax provides four grams of satiating fiber so be sure to keep those in the mix if you're looking to sip as much protein as possible.

7. Key Lime Pie Shake (42 g protein)

Nutrition: 212 calories, 0 g fat, 0 g sat fat, 17 g carbs, 0.7 g fiber, 7 g sugar, 42 g protein

Protein Source: Fat-free cottage cheese and protein powder

Key Lime pie may taste great, but with ingredients like heavy cream, sweetened condensed milk, butter, and sugar it's anything but great for your waistline. This shake, on the other hand, is low in sugar and overflowing with 42 grams of muscle-building protein—that's more than a day's worth of the nutrient for someone who's not very active and nearly half of what you'll need if you're a religious gym rat. We know the addition of cottage cheese may sound a bit strange, but that's what gives this drink its satisfying milkshake-esque consistency. If you're sensitive to dairy, swap in tofu to achieve the same texture. To keep your drink as healthy as possible, nix the pudding mix and xanthan gum—they only add calories and chemicals you don't need.

8. Skinny High Protein Oreo Milkshake (19 g protein)

Nutrition: 211 calories, 3.3 g fat, 0.9 g sat fat, 24 g carbs, 0 g fiber, 19 grams sugar, 19 grams protein

Protein Source: Cottage cheese, skim milk

Fat-free cottage cheese, skim milk, cookies, vanilla and a touch of Stevia team up to create a mouthwatering con-coction that only tastes sinful. While it is a bit high in sugar, 13 grams are the naturally occurring variety from the dairy, so it won't throw your diet off track. Although this drink shouldn't be your everyday go-to—it does contain Oreos, after all—it's an excellent alternative whenever a craving for something sweet strikes. Opting for this over a Dairy Queen Oreo Cookie Blizzard of the same size will save you 20 grams of fat and 48 grams of sugar!

9. Sunrise Smoothie (8 g protein)

Nutrition: 209 calories, 1.8 g fat, 0 g saturated fat, 42 g carbs, 6 g fiber, 28 g sugar 8 g protein

Protein Source: Greek yogurt

You'll be whisked away on a mini mental-vacation the second you start sipping this tropical-tasting smoothie. Don't let the high carb and sugar count scare you off; it's coming from berries, an orange and banana—all vitamin- and fiber-rich produce that will keep you trim and healthy.

10. Dark Chocolate Peppermint Shake (13 g protein)

Nutrition: 153 calories, 3.2 g fat, 0.9 g sat fat, 20 g carbs, 3 g fiber, 9 grams sugar, 13 grams protein (calculated with unsweetened almond milk)

Protein Source: Protein powder and optional Greek yogurt

This minty sweet shake allows you to enjoy the taste of Chocolate Peppermint Bark no matter what time of year it is—and without all the sugar and fat. It may taste like dessert, but thankfully, it doesn't have the same waist-expanding effects. Top your drink with a dollop of Greek yogurt to take the presentation and protein count to the next level.

11. Almond Butter Protein Smoothie (8 g protein)

Nutrition: 280 calories, 14 g fat, 1 g saturated fat, 39 g carbs, 9 g fiber, 17 g sugar, 7.5 g protein

Protein Source: Almond butter, chia seeds

Made with just four ingredients, this smoothie will take you no time at all to whip up. The almond milk and nut butter provide a solid hit of natural protein while the chia seeds lend a boost of antioxidants and heart-protecting omega-3s. Enjoy this as a healthy breakfast on the go or an afternoon snack. To kick your shake up a notch, add a few shakes of cinnamon. It will not only heighten the drink's taste, but also zap stubborn belly fat and help stabilize your blood sugar, which can ward off diet-derailing cravings.

12. Coffee Banana Protein Smoothie (10 g protein)
Serves: 3

Nutrition: 260 calories, 2 g fat, 0 g saturated fat, 50 g carbs, 6 g fiber, 34 g sugar, 10 g protein

Protein Source: Greek yogurt

What do yogurt, bananas, and coffee all have in common? They're all delicious breakfast go-to's that join together to create this energy-boosting protein smoothie. The mix of caffeine, natural sugar, and protein is ideal after a tough morning workout. If you're looking for a bit more protein or a thicker texture, add a bit more yogurt or some 2% milk.

13. Grape and Blueberry Protein Smoothie (9 g protein)
Nutrition: 320 calories, 9 g fat, 1.8 g saturated fat, 6.5 g fiber, 37 g sugar, 9 g protein

Protein Source: Cooked and cooled scrambled eggs

If you're not big into the idea of using nutrition powders —or you've simply run of out your go-to—you'll love this creative recipe. The blogger calls for a scrambled and blended egg in lieu of whey or plant protein, which is a fat-incinerating idea we totally love! The egg's protein aids muscle recovery and the choline in the yolk fights fat cells to give you that lean look you crave. As an added bonus, the berries and grapes provide more than a day's worth of vitamin C, which aids trim-down efforts further by warding off cortisol, a pesky stress hormone that triggers the storage of fat.

14. French Toast Protein Shake (42 g protein)
Nutrition: 235 calories, 0 g fat, 0 g sat fat, 12 g carbs, 1.2 g fiber, 14 g sugar, 42 g protein

Protein Source: Fat-free cottage cheese and protein powder

The fresh French toast taste you love with a lot more protein and a fraction of the fat and calories—now that's something worth waking up for! Though we love the idea of this shake, we're not so keen on the recommended three to five packets of Stevia. Since the sweetener is so much sweeter than sugar, we suggest starting with two packets and slowly adding more if you think it's needed. The less you can get away with using, the better.

15. Berry Oat Smoothie (11 g protein)
Nutrition: 280 calories, 4.9 g fat (2.3 g sat fat), 3.3 g fiber, 35.9 g sugar, 10.6 g protein

Protein Source: Milk, Greek yogurt

Sometimes you're just not in the mood for oatmeal, no matter how good it is for you. This smoothie blends plenty of antioxidant-rich blueberries with oats to ensure you still get the benefits and stay full all the way through to lunchtime. Just make sure you're using one of our best yogurts for weight loss in your at-home version.

16. Chocolate Peanut Butter Banana Breakfast Shake (11 g protein)

Nutrition: 346 calories, 19.2 g fat (4.2 g sat fat), 7.8 g fiber, 19.9 g sugar, 11.1 g protein

Protein Source: Peanut butter

Frozen bananas and peanut butter team up to give this smoothie a rich, milkshake-like consistency that will make you think it's sinful. When you use unsweetened almond milk, though, it's packed with protein without sky-high sugar counts found in other smoothies.

17. Blueberry Almond Butter Smoothie (18 g protein)

Nutrition: 585 calories, 37.8 g fat (4.1 g sat fat), 7.0 g fiber, 26.6 g sugar, 18.6 g protein

Protein Source: Almond butter, Greek yogurt

If you're looking for a meal-replacement smoothie, look no further. This one's overflowing with protein from rich almond butter and antioxidants from frozen blueberries. With over 18 grams of protein and a hefty dose of fiber, cravings won't come crawling back an hour later.

18. Raw Chocolate Smoothie (13 g protein)

Nutrition: 437 calories, 19.5 g fat (4.4 g sat fat), 11 g fiber, 34.7 g sugar, 12.4 g protein

Protein Source: Peanut butter

Raw cacao is different from that supermarket chocolate in two very important ways: it's packed with powerful antioxidants and boasts a surprisingly high amount of fiber. Paired with a portioned amount of honey, it's as sweet and indulgent as what you're used to, except it's actually good for you.

19. Raw Banana Bread Shakes (9 g protein)

Nutrition: 307 calories, 20.2 g fat (2 g sat fat), 6.9 g fiber, 12.6 g sugar, 9.3 g protein

Protein Source: Walnuts

You'll get all the warm, comforting flavor of the weekend breakfast staple without any of the flour or butter when you pick this smoothie. Plus, walnuts boast healthy omega-3s, protein, and fiber to keep you satiated.

20. Peach & Oat Breakfast Smoothie (11 g protein)

Per 1.7 cup serving: 263 calories, 3 g fat, 6 g fiber, 26 g sugars, 11 g protein (calculated with nonfat strawberry Greek yogurt and unsweetened almond milk)

Protein Source: Greek yogurt

Frozen peaches, ripe banana, fiber-filled oats, almond milk, and protein-packed Greek yogurt deliver a filling breakfast in just three minutes. With 11 grams of protein and 6 grams of fiber, it'll stave off the mid-morning hanger.

21. Carrot Cake Smoothie (10 g protein)

Per 1 cup serving: 219 calories, 13 g fat, 4 g fiber, 11 g sugars, 10 g protein (calculated with nonfat vanilla Greek yogurt, 1/2 cup of coconut and 1/2 cup of walnuts)

Protein Source: Greek yogurt

This carrot-cake smoothie is rich in healthy fats: Polyunsaturated fatty acids, like those in walnuts, may increase diet-induced calorie burn and resting metabolic rate. And walnuts have more heart healthy omega-3 fatty acids than any other nut! Bonus: One cup of this smoothie provides a day's worth of Vitamin A.

22. Orange Julius Protein Smoothie (16 g protein)

Nutrition: 130 calories, 2 g fat, 15 g carbs, 4 g fiber, 8 g sugar, 16 g protein

Protein Source: Low fat cottage cheese (or Greek yogurt)

The mall rat's favorite sugar bomb gets a healthy, protein-rich reboot. Cottage cheese (or Greek yogurt) provides a solid base of protein, and orange zest and juice impart sweetness and antioxidants without a surplus of sugar.

MOST COMMON PROTEIN SHAKE MISTAKES

Make sure your protein powder is working for you, not against

If you're looking to build muscle quickly, boost your macros and even shrink your recovery time, it's hard to beat a decent protein shake — whether whey or vegan. With research proving that protein supplementation, as part of a resistance training programme, can maintain lean body mass and increase strength, adding protein shakes to your diet quickly becomes a no-brainer if you're looking to build strength, size or athleticism.

But remember, with great amounts of protein comes great responsibility. It's important to know that protein supplementation isn't a catch-all solution for guys looking to add mass quickly. Rather, it's a convenient way of increasing your protein intake day-to-day and, for some, a solution to curbing a sweet tooth. There are, however, certain hurdles you should overcome to truly become a master of the protein shake.

It's not just average Joes tripping up, either. In fact, a study conducted by the University of Montreal found that three in four professional athletes failed to improve their performance or recovery with the help of protein shakes because they don't know how to take them properly. Thankfully, that needn't apply to you. Below, Men's Health walks you through your need-to-know guide.

PROTEIN: WHAT IS IT?

Firstly, let's go back to basics. If you know what you are actually consuming, then you are less likely to make mistakes. At its simplest, protein is a molecule made from chemicals called amino acids. Our bodies need these amino acids to function properly – they carry oxygen through blood, boost the immune system and build muscle.

There are 20 different amino acids in all, nine of which the human body can't produce. These are known as 'essential' amino acids and we need to get them from food.

SO, HOW MUCH PROTEIN DO I NEED?

It depends on your training goals. The US Food and Nutrition Board's current guidelines for the average adult is 0.8g of protein per kg of bodyweight. If you're looking to bulk up, you'll need to increase this number, but that's not as easy as simply stuffing your face.

You have to play it a bit smarter. Instead of reaching for calorie-dense foods, opt for high-protein foods. Not only will these cupboard staples build mass in your muscle groups — currently, research suggests, 2.2g of protein per kg of bodyweight is your limit — but also help stave off any hunger pangs that could derail even the most diligent of dieters.

For example, if you weigh 100kg, you'd need to be eating the equivalent of seven chicken breasts every day. Seven. A tad unrealistic. This type of extreme eating (and this amount) is reserved for competitive bodybuilders, so an achievable alternative for a first timer is 1.5g of protein per kg of bodyweight.

The amount you need to eat is a complex topic, and there is no one size fits all. It's important to tailor your intake to your workouts. Here's how to do it.

WHAT FOOD SHOULD I BE EATING?

It's vital that you realize protein shakes should never replace real foods. Ever. Protein shakes are supplements, and they are there to do just that — to supplement your diet. They are add-ons. Additional extras to help you reach your daily protein fix. Yes, we know, consuming a shed load of protein every day isn't easy. But it's important you don't cut corners.

Protein shakes will never hold the same nutritional benefits as real food, which will generally contain more protein per serving than a shake.

Whey Protein or Casein Protein? What's the Difference?

Right, you now know what you should be eating and have stocked your larder with high-protein foods. Next up: knowing is what is actually in your protein shake. Bear with us, your mistakes are coming. Quite simply, milk contains two main types of protein: whey and casein.

WHEY PROTEIN

Whey protein is found in the watery portion of milk and is a mixture of protein isolates. It's considered a complete protein – it contains all nine essential amino acids, which the body can't produce. That's why whey protein shakes are so important for muscle gain and why they are so popular in fitness circles. Generally, whey protein contains lower levels of fat and carbohydrates, minimizing gut distress and helps with weight-loss.

WHEY ISOLATE

So you know your casein from your whey protein, but do you know about whey isolate? Whey isolate, generally speaking, goes through more processing to eliminate reserves of fat, carbohydrates and lactose. Because of this, whey isolate is normally more expensive than regular whey protein.

CASEIN

Unlike whey, casein is a sl0w releasing protein, which can take up to six hours to completely digest and be utilized. Casein will help drip-feed your muscles over several hours, ensuring your body is constantly topped up with protein.

It's not ideal during the day – after a gym session – when your body desperately needs that protein fix. However, taking Casein last thing at night – the time when your body recovers best – is the most practical way to keep your muscles firing on all cylinders, avoiding 'starvation mode' – when your body starts to break down muscle for fuel.

If you want to fully maximize your fitness goals, then you will need to consume a combination of both casein and whey protein (although not in the same shake). A study conducted by Baylor University, Texas, observed 36 males undergoing heavy strength training and discovered that the group consuming a whey and casein combination far out-performed those who were on a combination of whey, BCAAs, and glutamine supplement. Over the 10-week period, results showed that those who took a combination of both protein supplements built significantly more lean muscle.

PROTEIN SHAKE MISTAKES YOU KEEP MAKING

So far, we've covered understanding what protein is, how protein shakes should never replace real food and how much protein you need to build muscle, plus the best sources. Read on for the mistakes you keep making.

Protein Shake Mistake #1: You're Overcomplicating Things

Got milk? Plus dried fruit and few scoops of almond butter? You're doing it wrong. Load up your DIY shake with too many ingredients and you're going to whack up the calorie count for no extra benefit.

The Fix

It's simple: opt for some low-sugar ingredients that will help you bulk up your muscle, not your belly. But where can you find recipes to shake up your protein plan? Good question: we've got some quick-to-make DIY shakes devised to help you build muscle all day long.

Protein Shake Mistake #2: You're Selling Yourself Short

When it comes to protein powder, there's no such thing as

cheap and cheerful. If your shake contains a concentrate powder with a suspiciously low price and a long shelf life then you're working out for something packed with fat and carbs. These are the best whey protein products you can buy.

The Fix

Whey Isolate protein. It's a touch more expensive, but when it comes to powder you get what you pay for. "Due to its long refinement processing, isolate will give you a higher quality protein without the unnecessary additives.

Not sure your current shake packs the right punch? Check one scoop of your powder contains at least 20-25 grams of protein. Drop below that and you'll soon notice your wallet shrinking and belly fat bulging.

Protein Shake Mistake #3: You've Gone Two Scoops Too Far

You really can have too much of a good thing. If you're filling your shopping basket to the brim with chicken and powder tubs then we've got some bad news: you're just going to the additional calories could just be increasing your waist line. In fact, trying to copy the diet of professional athletes will only set you up for a career in one sport: sumo wrestling.

The Fix

Calculators at the ready: you need (as we have mentioned) 1.5 to 2 grams of protein per kilo of bodyweight per day if you want to bulk up. This means if you're the UK average of 83kg, you need at least 133 grams of protein each day. Don't be put off if this sounds like a lot, as one chicken breast contains around 30g of protein. This means you can easily consume enough without resorting to sups. If you've already chowed down a protein-packed chicken salad for lunch and a bulk-up burger for dinner, chances are you've already met you protein requirements.

Protein Shake Mistake #4: You're making a Meal of It

There are too many guys who think all protein is created equal and are swapping for shakes. Don't be one of them. It might be quick to take, but a high calorie smoothie is unlikely to fill you up and won't give you as many nutrients as a proper meal. Plus, a full course means your body has to work harder to break down the food so you use up more calories in the digestion process.

The Fix

If your busy work day makes it too tempting to trade in a meal for a whey shake, then prep your lunchtime the night before. "Focus on things like fish, chicken, turkey, and beef for the best protein. They've got far more nutrients to keep you full. That's right, investing in some foil, Tupperware and a Mexican tuna salad could be a key step to a chiselled core.

Protein Shake Mistake #5: You're Neglecting the Little Guys

Cheap protein shake powder not only comes with an extra dose of carbs and fats, but also strips away the amino acids vital for muscle growth. Not only will you struggle to add size, you'll recover more slowly too. That means sore muscles putting the brakes on your performance.

The Fix

Keep your eyes peeled for two things: BCAAs and leucine.

A quality powder will be jammed with BCAAs (branched-chain amino acids) crucial for growth. And leucine? "It's is the key acid that stimulates muscle protein synthesis and growth. You need 3 grams of leucine to start this process always read the label.

Protein Shake Mistake #6: You've Got a One-shake Mind

Once you've invested in a massive tub of protein powder, it's only good for shakes, right? Wrong. Constricting yourself to mixing it with milk or water alone means you're missing out on more muscle building and tasty alternatives.

The Fix

Add it to your meals to get the protein you need, as well as the nutrients. And the earlier, the better. Research from the University of Missouri-Columbia found adding a scoop to your breakfast porridge or cinnamon pancakes will make you less likely to overeat during the day.

Protein Shake Mistake #7: Your Timing Is All Wrong

Before? During? A lot of men are wrongly led to believe by the Bro Science community that, as long as the protein is in your system, then you're sorted. However, when it comes to supps working out when to take them can be just as important as what you're taking.

The Fix

When is the best time for a shake? Within an hour after your workout. Because they're more receptive, this is the time to feed your muscles the fuel they need to repair and recover, leading to faster growth. If you're looking to prime yourself before a workout then don't rely on powder. This rustic spinach and pepper omelette, for instance, will give you the fuel for a full muscle-building session.

Protein Shake Mistake #8: Beware of Intolerance

A lot of protein powders will contain dairy, soy, corn starch, and additives your body may be unfamiliar with or allergic to. Whey is by far the most popular powdered protein and, if you have an issue with dairy, whey will have all the same problems being as it is, a milk derivative.

Soy protein isolate can be cheaply obtained and can cause inflammation, nausea and skin conditions. Corn starch has a habit of sending your blood sugar into peaks and troughs. Reading the long and complex ingredients list can be tough going but may just save your workout.

The Fix

While you're trying new shakes, keep a record of what you're taking and how you feel, so you can identify the culprit in the event of any unwanted side effects. Try to keep a food diary so you can monitor everything you're consuming. Listen to your body. Allergies make themselves known quickly so be aware of any changes in digestion and complexion.

There is still no substitute for hard work, a solid training plan and a proper nutrition routine. Supplements may make a little difference but unless you've nailed the first three, it's likely to be an exercise in futility.

Protein Shake Mistake #9: Getting Your Intake 'Window' Wrong

You don't need to inhale a four-egg omlette with a side of

whey protein as soon as you've completed your cooldown. According to a review published in the Journal of the International Society of Sports Nutrition, your muscle groups are primed for protein for a larger 'window' than previously thought. So you don't need to rush things as soon as you're out of the showers.

The Fix

While everybody is different, it's thought that timing your pre and post-exercise meals could be your greatest muscle-building ally if adding size is your primary goal. For example, if you start your day with a pre-gym snack at 7AM, you don't actually need another protein hit until your breakfast at 11AM. Your gains won't shrivel away and, if you're chasing strength and size, work to 0.7g to 1g of protein per pound of your bodyweight — a figure that's achievable if you split your macros across three to five meals in the day. Whether that's a protein shake or an egg white omelette, we'll leave that decision to you.

Sign up to the Men's Health newsletter and kickstart your home body plan. Make positive steps to become healthier and mentally strong with all the best fitness, muscle-building and nutrition advice delivered to your inbox.

CONCLUSION

Most people can easily get enough protein without using shakes. That being said, these supplements are an easy, safe and delicious way to add extra protein in your diet.

If you're trying to lose weight, extra protein from shakes can help you feel less hungry, help you lose weight faster and lower the likelihood of regaining the lost fat.